DIABETIC GASTROPARESIS DIET COOKBOOK FOR BEGINNERS

Are you in diabetic gastroparesis pain, get ready to stay fitness with this special recipes, +30day meal plan to nutrious your health today.

Dr. D. SAM

TABLE OF CONTENT

INTRODUCTION

Welcome to the ultimate guide for beginners navigating the challenges of diabetic gastroparesis. Our cookbook is designed to empower you on your journey to better health and well-being. Inside, you'll find a collection of carefully crafted recipes tailored to support your digestive system and manage blood sugar levels effectively. From hearty breakfasts to satisfying dinners and everything in between, each recipe is crafted with simplicity and taste in mind. Whether you're looking to kickstart your wellness journey or seeking inspiration for flavorful meals, this cookbook is your trusted companion. Let's embark on this culinary adventure together and embrace a deliciously fulfilling lifestyle. Get ready to savor every bite and take control of your health—one recipe at a time."

A disorder called diabetic gastroparesis affects the muscles in the stomach and makes it difficult for the stomach to empty properly. This particular form of neuropathy, or nerve damage, affects diabetics. For a more thorough explanation, see this:

The pathophysiological understanding

Nerve Damage: The vagus nerve, which regulates the passage of food through the digestive tract, is damaged in diabetic gastroparesis. Elevated blood sugar levels have the potential to alter the chemical composition of nerves and harm the blood vessels that supply the nerves with nutrition and oxygen.

Delayed Gastric Emptying: Food remains in the stomach for longer than usual because the stomach muscles are not contracting correctly. A number of digestive issues may result from this delay in stomach emptying.

Signs and symptoms

Vomiting and nausea are frequent symptoms brought on by the food moving slowly from the stomach into the small intestine.

Bloating: Having a full feeling, particularly after a modest meal.

Upper abdominal discomfort or pain is referred to as abdominal pain.

Malnutrition and weight loss: As a result of decreased appetite and inadequate food absorption.

Blood Sugar Fluctuations: The unpredictability of stomach emptying can lead to irregular blood glucose levels, which can make managing diabetes more difficult.

Gastric emptying study diagnosis: A test that gauges the amount of time it takes food to pass from the stomach into the small intestine.

Endoscopy: To exclude alternative reasons for the symptoms.

Measures the electrical and muscular activity of the stomach by gastric manometry.

Handling

Dietary Changes: To facilitate easier digestion, eat smaller, more frequent meals that are low in fat and fiber.

Medication: Prokinetic medicines (such as metoclopramide) to induce contractions of the stomach muscles; antiemetics to prevent nausea and vomiting.

Blood Sugar Management: Strict regulation of blood sugar levels to stop more nerve injury.

Gastric Electrical Stimulation: An implanted gadget that stimulates the stomach muscles with electrical pulses to assist manage nausea and vomiting.

Supervisory

Frequent follow-ups are necessary to track the disease's development and modify treatment plans as necessary.

Dietitian consultation is necessary to guarantee enough nutrition and control symptoms with food.

Hydration: Making sure you're getting enough fluids, particularly if you frequently experience vomiting.

Diabetic gastroparesis is a difficult condition to manage; endocrinologists, gastroenterologists, dietitians, and occasionally surgeons are involved in the multidisciplinary approach.

FOODS NOT TO EAT IN GASTROPARESIS DIABETICS

Making thoughtful food selections to facilitate digestion and keep blood sugar levels steady is essential to managing diabetic gastroparesis. Here are some foods to stay away from and the reasons you should cut them out of your diet:

High-Fat Foods: The slowing down of stomach emptying caused by fat can exacerbate symptoms.

Examples include fatty meat cuts, fried foods, fast food, heavy cream, butter, and high-fat snacks like cookies and chips.

Foods High in Fiber: Fiber can be problematic for digestion and can clog pipes, especially in the stomach when digestion is already sluggish.

Whole grains, unprocessed veggies, fruits with skins, beans, lentils, and legumes are a few examples.

Tough Foods to Digestion

Reason: Some foods are just more difficult to digest than others, which can lead to uncomfortable side effects like bloating.

Examples include fibrous vegetables like broccoli, corn, and cabbage, popcorn, hard meat cuts, and nuts and seeds.

Carbonated Drinks

Reason: Bloating and increased stomach discomfort can be brought on by carbonation.

Beer, soda, and sparkling water are a few examples.

High-Sugar Foods: Some of them may lead to delayed stomach emptying, and they can induce fast blood sugar rises that are problematic for managing diabetes.

Examples include sweetened beverages, desserts, sugary cereals, candies, and pastries.

Foods That Are Spicy: Spices have the potential to aggravate symptoms by irritating the stomach lining.

Spicy sauces, hot peppers, and highly spiced foods are a few examples.

Both caffeine and alcohol

Reason: Both may cause upset stomachs and have an impact on blood sugar levels.

Caffeinated sodas, coffee, energy drinks, and alcoholic beverages are among examples.

High-Fiber Supplements: These supplements might be hard to digest, much like high-fiber foods.

Examples include psyllium husk, bran, and meal replacements high in fiber.

Big Lunches

Reason: Eating a lot at once might cause the stomach to feel fuller longer and take longer to empty.

Plan: Choose to eat smaller, more frequent meals during the day.

Advice on Managing Your Diet

Foods that have been pureed or liquidized: These are frequently easier to digest and can support nutritional intake without aggravating symptoms.

Raw vegetables are more difficult to digest than cooked ones. De-seeding and peeling can also be beneficial.

Lean Proteins: Choose proteins that are simple to digest, such as eggs, fish, and chicken.

Low-Fat Dairy: To cut back on fat, go for non-fat or low-fat dairy products.

Smooth Foods: Digestion of foods such as mashed potatoes, yogurt, and applesauce may be facilitated.

Creating a meal plan with the assistance of a registered dietitian can help ensure that nutritional requirements are met and symptoms are adequately managed.

WHAT TO EAT WHEN YOU HAVE DIABETIC GASTROPARESIS

It's crucial to concentrate on foods that are simpler to digest, support stable blood sugar levels, and offer enough nourishment for those with diabetic gastroparesis. The following foods and dietary tips are available:

Simple to Digest Foods

Lean protein foods include tofu, eggs, fish, poultry, and turkey. They supply vital nutrients and are usually well-tolerated.

Low-Fat Dairy: cottage cheese, milk, yogurt, and low-fat cheese. These don't contribute much fat and can supply calcium and protein.

Low-Fiber Produce

Squash, carrots, zucchini, and green beans are examples of well-cooked vegetables since they are softer and simpler to digest.

Pureed veggies: Pumpkin and sweet potatoes are examples of mashed or pureed veggies.

Low-Fiber Fruits

Fruits that have been cooked or canned include applesauce, pears, peaches, and other skinless fruits.

Fruit juices: Isotonic varieties with no pulp are also a good choice, but use caution because of the high sugar content.

Clean Grains

Rice and white bread are easier to digest than complete grains.

Pasta: Particularly when it's cooked all the way through.

Pureed or Liquid Foods

Soups and broths: When pureed, they can be particularly easy to digest and nutritious.

Protein powder, low-fat yogurt, and low-fiber fruits are the ingredients of smoothies.

Replacement Meals Shakes: Made especially for those with gastroparesis, these can offer a well-balanced diet.

Good Fats

Tiny Amounts of Nutritious Fats: Smooth, not chunky nut butters, avocado, and olive oil (in moderation).

Small Meals Often

Approach: Throughout the day, eating smaller meals more regularly can help manage symptoms more effectively than bigger ones.

Cooking Techniques

Don't Fryer: To cut fat content, use baking, grilling, steaming, or boiling.

Foods can be made easier to digest by mashing or pureeing them.

Drinking Water

Keep Yourself Hydrated: Choose clear broths and herbal teas, and drink lots of water.

Protein powder: To guarantee a sufficient intake of protein, mix it into soups, smoothies, and other liquid meals.

Sample Menu

Breakfast is a smoothie made with bananas, low-fat yogurt, and a tiny bit of protein powder.

Applesauce or a tiny portion of low-fat cottage cheese would be a good mid-morning snack.

Lunch would be a pureed vegetable soup paired with tender, cooked chicken chunks.

Snack in the Afternoon: A piece of white bread spread with creamy peanut butter.

Dinner is baked fish served with perfectly cooked carrots and mashed potatoes.

Snack in the evening: A meal replacement shake or low-fat yogurt.

Advice on How to Prepare Meals

Blending and straining: To achieve the smoothest texture possible for smoothies and soups.

Fruits and vegetables should be peeled to lower the fiber content.

Observation and Modification

Frequent Check-Ins: To modify the diet in accordance with symptoms and nutritional requirements, see a nutritionist or healthcare professional.

Monitoring blood sugar involves keeping an eye on levels to make sure they stay constant.

By facilitating digestion and preserving nutritional balance, these dietary modifications can aid in the management of diabetic gastroparesis. For individualized nutritional planning, close collaboration with a medical professional or dietician is essential.

BREAKFAST RECIPES

1. Smooth Banana Yogurt Shake

Ingredients:

- 1 ripe banana

- 1 cup low-fat yogurt
- 1/2 cup low-fat milk or almond milk
- 1 tablespoon honey (optional, for added sweetness)
- 1 scoop protein powder (optional)

Instructions:

1. Peel the banana and cut it into small pieces.
2. Place the banana, yogurt, milk, and honey (if using) in a blender.
3. Add the protein powder if desired.
4. Blend until smooth.
5. Pour into a glass and serve immediately.

2. Scrambled Eggs with Cheese

Ingredients:

- 2 large eggs
- 2 tablespoons low-fat milk
- 1/4 cup shredded low-fat cheese (such as cheddar or mozzarella)
- Salt and pepper to taste

- 1 teaspoon olive oil or cooking spray

Instructions:

1. In a bowl, whisk the eggs and milk together until well combined.
2. Heat the olive oil in a non-stick skillet over medium heat.
3. Pour the egg mixture into the skillet.
4. Cook, stirring frequently, until the eggs are almost set.
5. Add the cheese and continue to cook until the eggs are fully set and the cheese is melted.
6. Season with salt and pepper to taste and serve.

3. Creamy Oatmeal

Ingredients:

- 1/2 cup quick-cooking oats
- 1 cup low-fat milk or almond milk
- 1/2 ripe banana, mashed
- 1 tablespoon smooth peanut butter

- 1 teaspoon honey or maple syrup (optional)

Instructions:

1. In a small saucepan, bring the milk to a boil.
2. Add the oats and reduce the heat to a simmer.
3. Cook, stirring frequently, for about 5 minutes or until the oats are soft and creamy.
4. Stir in the mashed banana and peanut butter.
5. Sweeten with honey or maple syrup if desired.
6. Serve warm.

4. Applesauce Pancakes

Ingredients:

- 1/2 cup all-purpose flour
- 1/2 teaspoon baking powder
- 1/4 teaspoon baking soda
- 1/4 teaspoon salt

- 1/2 cup unsweetened applesauce
- 1/4 cup low-fat milk or almond milk
- 1 large egg
- 1 teaspoon vanilla extract
- Cooking spray

Instructions:

1. In a bowl, whisk together the flour, baking powder, baking soda, and salt.
2. In another bowl, combine the applesauce, milk, egg, and vanilla extract.
3. Add the wet ingredients to the dry ingredients and stir until just combined.
4. Heat a non-stick skillet or griddle over medium heat and lightly coat with cooking spray.
5. Pour 1/4 cup of the batter onto the skillet for each pancake.
6. Cook until bubbles form on the surface and the edges look set, then flip and cook until golden brown.

7. Serve warm with a small amount of syrup or fruit puree.

5. Cottage Cheese and Fruit Bowl

Ingredients:

- 1 cup low-fat cottage cheese
- 1/2 cup canned peaches or pears (packed in juice or water, not syrup), drained and diced
- 1 tablespoon honey or agave nectar (optional)
- A sprinkle of cinnamon (optional)

Instructions:

1. Spoon the cottage cheese into a bowl.
2. Top with the diced peaches or pears.
3. Drizzle with honey or agave nectar if desired.
4. Sprinkle with cinnamon for extra flavor.
5. Serve immediately.

6. Spinach and Feta Omelette

Ingredients:

- 2 large eggs
- 2 tablespoons low-fat milk
- 1/4 cup fresh spinach, finely chopped
- 2 tablespoons crumbled feta cheese
- Salt and pepper to taste
- 1 teaspoon olive oil or cooking spray

Instructions:

1. In a bowl, whisk together the eggs and milk until well combined.
2. Heat the olive oil in a non-stick skillet over medium heat.
3. Pour the egg mixture into the skillet and cook until the edges start to set.
4. Sprinkle the chopped spinach and feta cheese over one half of the omelette.
5. Fold the omelette in half and continue to cook until fully set.
6. Season with salt and pepper to taste and serve.

7. Vanilla Rice Pudding

Ingredients:

- 1/2 cup cooked white rice
- 1 cup low-fat milk or almond milk
- 1 tablespoon honey or agave nectar
- 1/2 teaspoon vanilla extract
- Ground cinnamon for garnish (optional)

Instructions:

1. In a small saucepan, combine the cooked rice and milk.
2. Cook over medium heat, stirring frequently, until the mixture thickens and becomes creamy (about 10-15 minutes).
3. Stir in the honey and vanilla extract.
4. Transfer to a bowl and sprinkle with ground cinnamon if desired.
5. Serve warm or chilled.

8. Pumpkin Smoothie

Ingredients:

- 1/2 cup canned pumpkin puree
- 1 cup low-fat milk or almond milk
- 1/2 ripe banana
- 1 tablespoon smooth almond butter
- 1/2 teaspoon ground cinnamon
- 1/4 teaspoon ground nutmeg
- 1 tablespoon honey or maple syrup (optional)

Instructions:

1. Place all ingredients in a blender.
2. Blend until smooth and creamy.
3. Pour into a glass and serve immediately.

9. Blueberry Yogurt Parfait

Ingredients:

- 1 cup low-fat Greek yogurt
- 1/2 cup fresh or thawed frozen blueberries
- 2 tablespoons granola (low-fat, low-sugar)
- 1 teaspoon honey (optional)

Instructions:

1. In a serving glass or bowl, layer half of the yogurt, followed by half of the blueberries and granola.
2. Repeat the layers with the remaining yogurt, blueberries, and granola.
3. Drizzle with honey if desired.
4. Serve immediately.

10. Soft Polenta with Honey

Ingredients:

- 1/4 cup quick-cooking polenta
- 1 cup low-fat milk or almond milk
- 1 tablespoon honey
- 1/4 teaspoon vanilla extract
- A pinch of salt

Instructions:

1. In a small saucepan, bring the milk to a boil.
2. Slowly whisk in the polenta and reduce the heat to low.

3. Cook, stirring constantly, until the polenta thickens (about 5 minutes).
4. Remove from heat and stir in the honey, vanilla extract, and salt.
5. Transfer to a bowl and serve warm.

1. Chicken and Vegetable Soup

Ingredients:

- 1 boneless, skinless chicken breast, diced
- 1 cup low-sodium chicken broth
- 1/2 cup carrots, peeled and diced
- 1/2 cup zucchini, diced
- 1/2 cup peeled and diced potatoes
- Salt and pepper to taste
- 1 teaspoon olive oil

Instructions:

1. Heat olive oil in a large pot over medium heat.

2. Add the diced chicken breast and cook until browned and cooked through.
3. Add the chicken broth, carrots, zucchini, and potatoes.
4. Bring to a boil, then reduce heat and simmer for about 20 minutes, or until the vegetables are tender.
5. Season with salt and pepper to taste.
6. Serve warm.

2. Turkey and Spinach Wrap

Ingredients:

- 1 whole wheat tortilla (soft and easy to digest)
- 3-4 slices of deli turkey (low sodium)
- 1/2 cup fresh spinach leaves
- 1/4 cup shredded low-fat cheese (such as mozzarella)
- 1 tablespoon low-fat mayonnaise or Greek yogurt
- 1 teaspoon Dijon mustard

Instructions:

1. Lay the tortilla flat on a plate.
2. Spread the mayonnaise or Greek yogurt and Dijon mustard over the tortilla.
3. Layer the turkey slices evenly over the tortilla.
4. Add the spinach leaves and shredded cheese on top of the turkey.
5. Roll the tortilla tightly into a wrap.
6. Slice in half and serve.

3. Baked Salmon with Mashed Sweet Potatoes

Ingredients:

- 1 salmon fillet (4-6 ounces)
- 1 medium sweet potato
- 1 teaspoon olive oil
- Salt and pepper to taste
- 1 teaspoon lemon juice
- 1 teaspoon chopped fresh parsley (optional)

Instructions:

1. Preheat the oven to 375°F (190°C).
2. Place the salmon fillet on a baking sheet lined with parchment paper.
3. Drizzle with olive oil and lemon juice, and season with salt and pepper.
4. Bake for 15-20 minutes, or until the salmon is cooked through and flakes easily with a fork.
5. While the salmon is baking, peel and dice the sweet potato.
6. Boil the sweet potato in a pot of water until tender, about 10-15 minutes.
7. Drain and mash the sweet potato until smooth.
8. Season with a little salt and pepper.
9. Serve the salmon alongside the mashed sweet potatoes, garnished with parsley if desired.

4. Quinoa and Vegetable Salad

Ingredients:

- 1/2 cup cooked quinoa
- 1/2 cup cherry tomatoes, halved

- 1/2 cup cucumber, diced
- 1/4 cup crumbled feta cheese
- 2 tablespoons olive oil
- 1 tablespoon lemon juice
- Salt and pepper to taste
- 1 tablespoon chopped fresh basil or parsley

Instructions:

1. In a large bowl, combine the cooked quinoa, cherry tomatoes, cucumber, and crumbled feta cheese.
2. In a small bowl, whisk together the olive oil, lemon juice, salt, and pepper.
3. Pour the dressing over the quinoa mixture and toss to combine.
4. Garnish with chopped basil or parsley.
5. Serve immediately or refrigerate until ready to eat.

5. Egg Salad Sandwich

Ingredients:

- 2 hard-boiled eggs, chopped

- 2 tablespoons low-fat mayonnaise or Greek yogurt
- 1 teaspoon Dijon mustard
- 1 teaspoon chopped fresh chives or green onion
- Salt and pepper to taste
- 2 slices soft whole wheat bread (crust removed if needed)

Instructions:

1. In a bowl, combine the chopped hard-boiled eggs, mayonnaise or Greek yogurt, Dijon mustard, and chopped chives or green onion.
2. Mix until well combined and season with salt and pepper to taste.
3. Spread the egg salad evenly over one slice of bread.
4. Top with the other slice of bread to form a sandwich.
5. Slice the sandwich in half and serve.

6. Chicken and Rice Casserole

Ingredients:

- 1 cup cooked white rice
- 1 cup cooked, shredded chicken breast
- 1/2 cup low-fat cream of chicken soup
- 1/4 cup low-fat milk
- 1/2 cup finely chopped carrots (cooked until soft)
- 1/2 cup finely chopped zucchini (cooked until soft)
- 1/4 cup shredded low-fat cheese
- Salt and pepper to taste

Instructions:

1. Preheat the oven to 350°F (175°C).
2. In a large bowl, combine the cooked rice, shredded chicken, cream of chicken soup, milk, carrots, and zucchini.
3. Mix until well combined and season with salt and pepper to taste.
4. Transfer the mixture to a lightly greased baking dish.
5. Sprinkle the shredded cheese on top.

6. Bake for 20-25 minutes, or until the casserole is heated through and the cheese is melted.
7. Serve warm.

7. Creamy Tomato Basil Soup

Ingredients:

- 1 can (14.5 ounces) diced tomatoes (no salt added)
- 1 cup low-sodium chicken or vegetable broth
- 1/2 cup low-fat milk or cream
- 1 tablespoon olive oil
- 1 small onion, finely chopped
- 1 clove garlic, minced
- 1/4 cup chopped fresh basil
- Salt and pepper to taste

Instructions:

1. Heat the olive oil in a large pot over medium heat.
2. Add the chopped onion and garlic and cook until softened, about 5 minutes.

3. Add the diced tomatoes and broth, and bring to a boil.
4. Reduce the heat and simmer for 15 minutes.
5. Use an immersion blender to puree the soup until smooth (or carefully transfer to a blender and blend in batches).
6. Stir in the milk or cream and chopped basil.
7. Season with salt and pepper to taste.
8. Serve warm.

8. Baked Tilapia with Mashed Cauliflower

Ingredients:

- 1 tilapia fillet (4-6 ounces)
- 1 teaspoon olive oil
- Salt and pepper to taste
- 1/2 teaspoon dried dill (optional)
- 1 small head cauliflower, chopped
- 1/4 cup low-fat milk or chicken broth
- 1 tablespoon butter or margarine

Instructions:

1. Preheat the oven to 375°F (190°C).
2. Place the tilapia fillet on a baking sheet lined with parchment paper.
3. Drizzle with olive oil and season with salt, pepper, and dill if using.
4. Bake for 15-20 minutes, or until the fish is cooked through and flakes easily with a fork.
5. Meanwhile, steam the cauliflower until tender, about 10-12 minutes.
6. Transfer the cauliflower to a blender or food processor, add the milk or broth and butter, and blend until smooth.
7. Season with salt and pepper to taste.
8. Serve the tilapia alongside the mashed cauliflower.

9. Turkey and Avocado Roll-Ups

Ingredients:

- 4 slices deli turkey (low sodium)
- 1/2 ripe avocado, sliced

- 1/4 cup shredded low-fat cheese (such as cheddar or mozzarella)
- 1 tablespoon low-fat mayonnaise or Greek yogurt
- 1 teaspoon lemon juice
- Salt and pepper to taste

Instructions:

1. Lay the turkey slices flat on a plate.
2. In a small bowl, mix the avocado slices with the lemon juice, and season with salt and pepper.
3. Spread the mayonnaise or Greek yogurt over the turkey slices.
4. Place a few slices of avocado on each turkey slice.
5. Sprinkle with shredded cheese.
6. Roll up each turkey slice tightly.
7. Secure with toothpicks if needed and serve.

10. Cottage Cheese and Cucumber Salad

Ingredients:

- 1 cup low-fat cottage cheese
- 1/2 cup cucumber, peeled, seeded, and finely chopped
- 1/4 cup diced tomatoes (seeds removed)
- 1 tablespoon chopped fresh dill or parsley
- 1 teaspoon lemon juice
- Salt and pepper to taste

Instructions:

1. In a bowl, combine the cottage cheese, cucumber, tomatoes, and chopped dill or parsley.
2. Add the lemon juice and mix well.
3. Season with salt and pepper to taste.
4. Serve chilled.

DINNER RECIPES

1. Lemon Herb Chicken with Steamed Green Beans

Ingredients:

- 1 boneless, skinless chicken breast
- 1 tablespoon olive oil
- 1 tablespoon lemon juice
- 1 teaspoon dried oregano
- 1 teaspoon dried basil
- Salt and pepper to taste
- 1 cup green beans, trimmed

Instructions:

1. Preheat the oven to 375°F (190°C).
2. In a small bowl, mix the olive oil, lemon juice, oregano, basil, salt, and pepper.
3. Place the chicken breast on a baking sheet lined with parchment paper.
4. Brush the lemon herb mixture over the chicken breast.
5. Bake for 25-30 minutes, or until the chicken is cooked through and juices run clear.

6. While the chicken is baking, steam the green beans until tender, about 5-7 minutes.
7. Serve the chicken breast alongside the steamed green beans.

2. Baked Cod with Mashed Carrots

Ingredients:

- 1 cod fillet (4-6 ounces)
- 1 teaspoon olive oil
- Salt and pepper to taste
- 1/2 teaspoon dried dill (optional)
- 2 large carrots, peeled and chopped
- 1 tablespoon butter or margarine
- 1/4 cup low-fat milk or chicken broth

Instructions:

1. Preheat the oven to 375°F (190°C).
2. Place the cod fillet on a baking sheet lined with parchment paper.
3. Drizzle with olive oil and season with salt, pepper, and dill if using.

4. Bake for 15-20 minutes, or until the fish is cooked through and flakes easily with a fork.
5. Meanwhile, steam the carrots until tender, about 10-12 minutes.
6. Transfer the carrots to a blender or food processor, add the butter and milk or broth, and blend until smooth.
7. Season with salt and pepper to taste.
8. Serve the cod alongside the mashed carrots.

3. Ground Turkey and Zucchini Skillet

Ingredients:

- 1/2 pound ground turkey
- 1 medium zucchini, diced
- 1 small onion, finely chopped
- 1 clove garlic, minced
- 1 tablespoon olive oil
- 1/2 cup low-sodium chicken broth
- 1/2 teaspoon dried thyme
- Salt and pepper to taste

Instructions:

1. Heat the olive oil in a large skillet over medium heat.
2. Add the chopped onion and minced garlic, and sauté until softened, about 5 minutes.
3. Add the ground turkey and cook until browned and cooked through, breaking it up with a spoon.
4. Add the diced zucchini, chicken broth, thyme, salt, and pepper.
5. Cook, stirring occasionally, until the zucchini is tender and the liquid has reduced, about 10 minutes.
6. Serve warm.

4. Soft Beef Tacos

Ingredients:

- 1/2 pound lean ground beef
- 1 small onion, finely chopped
- 1 clove garlic, minced
- 1/2 cup low-sodium beef broth

- 1 teaspoon ground cumin
- 1/2 teaspoon paprika
- Salt and pepper to taste
- 4 small soft flour tortillas
- 1/2 cup shredded lettuce
- 1/4 cup shredded low-fat cheese (such as cheddar or mozzarella)
- 1/4 cup diced tomatoes (seeds removed)

Instructions:

1. Heat a large skillet over medium heat and add the ground beef, chopped onion, and minced garlic.
2. Cook until the beef is browned and the onion is softened, about 7-10 minutes.
3. Add the beef broth, cumin, paprika, salt, and pepper.
4. Simmer for about 5 minutes, or until the liquid has reduced.
5. Warm the flour tortillas in a dry skillet or microwave.

6. Fill each tortilla with the beef mixture, shredded lettuce, cheese, and diced tomatoes.
7. Serve immediately.

5. Vegetable and Tofu Stir-Fry

Ingredients:

- 1/2 block firm tofu, drained and cubed
- 1 cup broccoli florets
- 1/2 cup sliced carrots
- 1/2 cup snow peas
- 1/4 cup low-sodium soy sauce
- 1 tablespoon olive oil
- 1 clove garlic, minced
- 1 teaspoon grated fresh ginger
- 1/4 cup low-sodium vegetable broth
- 1 teaspoon cornstarch mixed with 1 tablespoon water (optional, for thickening)

Instructions:

1. Heat the olive oil in a large skillet or wok over medium heat.

2. Add the minced garlic and grated ginger, and sauté for about 1 minute.
3. Add the cubed tofu and cook until lightly browned on all sides.
4. Add the broccoli, carrots, and snow peas to the skillet.
5. Stir-fry for about 5-7 minutes, or until the vegetables are tender-crisp.
6. Add the soy sauce and vegetable broth, and stir to combine.
7. If using, add the cornstarch mixture and cook until the sauce has thickened.
8. Serve warm.

6. Shrimp and Rice Bowl

Ingredients:

- 1 cup cooked white rice
- 1/2 pound shrimp, peeled and deveined
- 1 tablespoon olive oil
- 1 clove garlic, minced
- 1/2 cup diced zucchini

- 1/2 cup diced bell pepper (optional, based on tolerance)
- 1 tablespoon low-sodium soy sauce
- 1 tablespoon lemon juice
- Salt and pepper to taste

Instructions:

1. Heat the olive oil in a large skillet over medium heat.
2. Add the minced garlic and cook until fragrant, about 1 minute.
3. Add the shrimp and cook until pink and opaque, about 2-3 minutes per side.
4. Remove the shrimp from the skillet and set aside.
5. Add the zucchini and bell pepper to the skillet and cook until tender, about 5-7 minutes.
6. Return the shrimp to the skillet and add the soy sauce and lemon juice.
7. Stir to combine and heat through.
8. Serve the shrimp and vegetable mixture over the cooked rice.

7. Chicken and Butternut Squash Puree

Ingredients:

- 1 boneless, skinless chicken breast
- 1 cup butternut squash, peeled and cubed
- 1 tablespoon olive oil
- 1/2 teaspoon dried thyme
- Salt and pepper to taste
- 1/4 cup low-sodium chicken broth

Instructions:

1. Preheat the oven to 375°F (190°C).
2. Place the chicken breast on a baking sheet lined with parchment paper.
3. Drizzle with olive oil and season with thyme, salt, and pepper.
4. Bake for 25-30 minutes, or until the chicken is cooked through and juices run clear.
5. Meanwhile, steam the butternut squash until tender, about 15-20 minutes.

6. Transfer the cooked squash to a blender or food processor, add the chicken broth, and blend until smooth.
7. Season the puree with salt and pepper to taste.
8. Serve the chicken breast alongside the butternut squash puree.

8. Baked Turkey Meatballs with Mashed Potatoes

Ingredients:

- 1/2 pound ground turkey
- 1/4 cup breadcrumbs (preferably whole wheat)
- 1 egg
- 1/4 cup grated Parmesan cheese
- 1 teaspoon dried Italian seasoning
- Salt and pepper to taste
- 2 medium potatoes, peeled and diced
- 1/4 cup low-fat milk or chicken broth
- 1 tablespoon butter or margarine

Instructions:

1. Preheat the oven to 375°F (190°C).
2. In a large bowl, combine the ground turkey, breadcrumbs, egg, Parmesan cheese, Italian seasoning, salt, and pepper.
3. Mix until well combined and form into small meatballs.
4. Place the meatballs on a baking sheet lined with parchment paper.
5. Bake for 20-25 minutes, or until the meatballs are cooked through.
6. Meanwhile, boil the diced potatoes in a pot of water until tender, about 15-20 minutes.
7. Drain the potatoes and mash them with the milk or chicken broth and butter until smooth.
8. Season with salt and pepper to taste.
9. Serve the meatballs alongside the mashed potatoes.

9. Mild Fish Curry

Ingredients:

- 1 white fish fillet (such as cod or tilapia), cut into chunks
- 1 tablespoon olive oil
- 1/2 small onion, finely chopped
- 1 clove garlic, minced
- 1/2 cup low-sodium chicken broth
- 1/2 cup canned coconut milk (light)
- 1 teaspoon ground turmeric
- 1/2 teaspoon ground cumin
- 1/4 teaspoon ground coriander
- Salt and pepper to taste
- 1/2 cup cooked white rice

Instructions:

1. Heat the olive oil in a large skillet over medium heat.
2. Add the chopped onion and minced garlic and cook until softened, about 5 minutes.
3. Add the turmeric, cumin, and coriander and cook for another 1-2 minutes.

4. Pour in the chicken broth and coconut milk, stirring to combine.
5. Add the fish chunks and simmer gently until the fish is cooked through, about 8-10 minutes.
6. Season with salt and pepper to taste.
7. Serve the fish curry over the cooked white rice.

10. Tofu and Carrot Ginger Soup

Ingredients:

- 1/2 block firm tofu, cubed
- 2 large carrots, peeled and diced
- 1 small onion, finely chopped
- 1 tablespoon olive oil
- 1 clove garlic, minced
- 1 teaspoon grated fresh ginger
- 3 cups low-sodium vegetable broth
- Salt and pepper to taste
- 1 tablespoon chopped fresh cilantro (optional)

Instructions:

1. Heat the olive oil in a large pot over medium heat.
2. Add the chopped onion, garlic, and grated ginger and cook until softened, about 5 minutes.
3. Add the diced carrots and vegetable broth.
4. Bring to a boil, then reduce the heat and simmer until the carrots are tender, about 15-20 minutes.
5. Use an immersion blender to puree the soup until smooth (or carefully transfer to a blender and blend in batches).
6. Add the cubed tofu and heat through.
7. Season with salt and pepper to taste.
8. Garnish with chopped fresh cilantro if desired.
9. Serve warm.

1. Greek Yogurt with Berries

Ingredients:

- 1/2 cup low-fat Greek yogurt
- 1/4 cup fresh berries (such as strawberries, blueberries, or raspberries)
- 1 tablespoon chopped nuts (such as almonds or walnuts) (optional)
- 1 teaspoon honey or agave nectar (optional)

Instructions:

1. Spoon the Greek yogurt into a bowl.
2. Top with fresh berries and chopped nuts if using.
3. Drizzle with honey or agave nectar if desired.
4. Serve immediately.

2. Cottage Cheese and Pineapple

Ingredients:

- 1/2 cup low-fat cottage cheese
- 1/4 cup diced pineapple (fresh or canned in juice)

- 1 tablespoon shredded coconut (optional)

Instructions:

1. Spoon the cottage cheese into a bowl.
2. Top with diced pineapple and shredded coconut if using.
3. Serve chilled.

3. Banana Peanut Butter Roll-Ups

Ingredients:

- 1 small banana
- 1 tablespoon smooth peanut butter
- 1 small whole wheat tortilla

Instructions:

1. Spread the peanut butter evenly over the whole wheat tortilla.
2. Place the banana on one edge of the tortilla.
3. Roll up the tortilla tightly around the banana.
4. Slice into bite-sized pieces and serve.

4. Veggie Sticks with Hummus

Ingredients:

- 1/2 cup baby carrots
- 1/2 cup cucumber sticks
- 1/4 cup cherry tomatoes
- 2 tablespoons hummus

Instructions:

1. Arrange the baby carrots, cucumber sticks, and cherry tomatoes on a plate.
2. Serve with hummus for dipping.

5. Apple Slices with Almond Butter

Ingredients:

- 1 small apple, sliced
- 1 tablespoon almond butter

Instructions:

1. Arrange the apple slices on a plate.
2. Serve with almond butter for dipping.

6. Hard-Boiled Eggs with Whole Grain Crackers

Ingredients:

- 2 hard-boiled eggs
- 4 whole grain crackers

Instructions:

1. Peel the hard-boiled eggs and slice them in half.
2. Serve with whole grain crackers on the side.

7. Avocado Rice Cakes

Ingredients:

- 1 rice cake
- 1/4 ripe avocado, mashed
- 1 teaspoon lemon juice
- Pinch of salt and pepper
- Optional toppings: sliced cherry tomatoes, cucumber, or radishes

Instructions:

1. Spread the mashed avocado on the rice cake.
2. Drizzle with lemon juice and season with salt and pepper.
3. Add optional toppings if desired.
4. Serve immediately.

8. Cottage Cheese with Sliced Peaches

Ingredients:

- 1/2 cup low-fat cottage cheese
- 1/2 fresh peach, sliced
- Sprinkle of cinnamon (optional)

Instructions:

1. Spoon the cottage cheese into a bowl.
2. Top with sliced peaches.
3. Sprinkle with cinnamon if desired.
4. Serve chilled.

9. Turkey and Cheese Roll-Ups

Ingredients:

- 2 slices low-sodium deli turkey

- 2 slices low-fat cheese (such as cheddar or Swiss)
- 1/4 cup baby spinach leaves

Instructions:

1. Lay one slice of turkey flat on a plate.
2. Place a slice of cheese and a few spinach leaves on top.
3. Roll up the turkey slice tightly.
4. Repeat with the remaining turkey, cheese, and spinach.
5. Slice the rolled-up turkey into bite-sized pieces and serve.

10. Tuna Salad Lettuce Wraps

Ingredients:

- 1 can (5 ounces) tuna, drained
- 1 tablespoon low-fat mayonnaise or Greek yogurt
- 1 teaspoon Dijon mustard
- 1/4 cup diced celery
- 1 tablespoon diced red onion
- Salt and pepper to taste

- 4 large lettuce leaves

Instructions:

1. In a bowl, combine the tuna, mayonnaise or Greek yogurt, Dijon mustard, celery, and red onion.
2. Mix until well combined and season with salt and pepper to taste.
3. Spoon the tuna salad onto the lettuce leaves.
4. Roll up the lettuce leaves to form wraps.
5. Serve immediately.

DESSERT RECIPES

1. Baked Apples with Cinnamon

Ingredients:

- 2 medium-sized apples
- 1 teaspoon cinnamon
- 1 tablespoon chopped nuts (such as walnuts or almonds) (optional)

- 1 teaspoon honey or agave nectar (optional)

Instructions:

1. Preheat the oven to 375°F (190°C).
2. Core the apples and place them in a baking dish.
3. Sprinkle cinnamon evenly over the apples.
4. If using, fill the center of each apple with chopped nuts and drizzle with honey or agave nectar.
5. Bake for 20-25 minutes, or until the apples are tender.
6. Serve warm.

2. Greek Yogurt with Honey and Almonds

Ingredients:

- 1/2 cup low-fat Greek yogurt
- 1 tablespoon honey
- 1 tablespoon sliced almonds

Instructions:

1. Spoon the Greek yogurt into a bowl.
2. Drizzle honey over the yogurt.
3. Sprinkle sliced almonds on top.
4. Serve immediately.

3. Berry Parfait

Ingredients:

- 1/2 cup low-fat cottage cheese
- 1/4 cup fresh berries (such as strawberries, blueberries, or raspberries)
- 1 tablespoon chopped nuts (such as almonds or walnuts) (optional)
- 1 teaspoon honey or agave nectar (optional)

Instructions:

1. In a glass or bowl, layer the cottage cheese and fresh berries.
2. If using, sprinkle chopped nuts over the berries.

3. Drizzle with honey or agave nectar if desired.
4. Serve chilled.

4. Cocoa Banana Smoothie

Ingredients:

- 1 ripe banana
- 1 tablespoon unsweetened cocoa powder
- 1/2 cup low-fat milk or almond milk
- 1/4 teaspoon vanilla extract
- 1 teaspoon honey or agave nectar (optional)
- Ice cubes (optional)

Instructions:

1. Peel the banana and place it in a blender.
2. Add the cocoa powder, milk, vanilla extract, and honey or agave nectar if using.
3. If desired, add a few ice cubes to the blender for a colder smoothie.

4. Blend until smooth and creamy.
5. Pour into a glass and serve immediately.

5. Chia Seed Pudding with Berries

Ingredients:

- 2 tablespoons chia seeds
- 1/2 cup low-fat milk or almond milk
- 1/4 teaspoon vanilla extract
- 1 teaspoon honey or agave nectar (optional)
- 1/4 cup fresh berries (such as strawberries, blueberries, or raspberries)

Instructions:

1. In a bowl, mix together the chia seeds, milk, vanilla extract, and honey or agave nectar if using.
2. Cover and refrigerate for at least 2 hours, or overnight, until the pudding thickens.
3. Stir the pudding well before serving.

4. Serve topped with fresh berries.

6. Peanut Butter Banana Bites

Ingredients:

- 1 ripe banana, sliced
- 2 tablespoons natural peanut butter
- 1 tablespoon unsweetened shredded coconut (optional)
- 1 tablespoon chopped nuts (such as almonds or walnuts) (optional)

Instructions:

1. Spread peanut butter on each banana slice.
2. Sprinkle with shredded coconut and chopped nuts if desired.
3. Serve immediately.

7. Vanilla Yogurt with Sliced Peaches

Ingredients:

- 1/2 cup low-fat vanilla yogurt
- 1/2 fresh peach, sliced

- 1 tablespoon granola (optional)

Instructions:

1. Spoon the vanilla yogurt into a bowl.
2. Top with sliced peaches.
3. Sprinkle granola over the peaches if desired.
4. Serve chilled.

8. Cinnamon Baked Pears

Ingredients:

- 2 medium pears, halved and cored
- 1/2 teaspoon cinnamon
- 1 tablespoon chopped nuts (such as walnuts or almonds) (optional)
- 1 teaspoon honey or agave nectar (optional)

Instructions:

1. Preheat the oven to 375°F (190°C).
2. Place the pear halves in a baking dish, cut side up.

3. Sprinkle cinnamon evenly over the pears.
4. If using, fill the center of each pear half with chopped nuts and drizzle with honey or agave nectar.
5. Bake for 20-25 minutes, or until the pears are tender.
6. Serve warm.

9. Strawberry Frozen Yogurt Bark

Ingredients:

- 1 cup low-fat Greek yogurt
- 1/2 cup sliced strawberries
- 1 tablespoon honey or agave nectar (optional)
- 1 tablespoon unsweetened shredded coconut (optional)

Instructions:

1. Line a baking sheet with parchment paper.

2. Spread the Greek yogurt evenly onto the parchment paper, about 1/4 inch thick.

3. Sprinkle sliced strawberries over the yogurt.

4. Drizzle with honey or agave nectar if desired.

5. If using, sprinkle shredded coconut over the top.

6. Place the baking sheet in the freezer for at least 2 hours, or until the yogurt bark is firm.

7. Break the bark into pieces and serve immediately.

10. Chilled Chocolate Avocado Pudding

Ingredients:

- 1 ripe avocado
- 2 tablespoons unsweetened cocoa powder
- 2 tablespoons honey or agave nectar
- 1/4 cup low-fat milk or almond milk

- 1/2 teaspoon vanilla extract
- Pinch of salt

Instructions:

1. Scoop the avocado flesh into a blender or food processor.
2. Add the cocoa powder, honey or agave nectar, milk, vanilla extract, and salt.
3. Blend until smooth and creamy.
4. Refrigerate for at least 30 minutes before serving.
5. Serve chilled.

Certainly! Here are five

DESSERT RECIPES

1. Baked Apples with Cinnamon

Ingredients:

- 2 medium-sized apples
- 1 teaspoon cinnamon
- 1 tablespoon chopped nuts (such as walnuts or almonds) (optional)

- 1 teaspoon honey or agave nectar (optional)

Instructions:

1. Preheat the oven to 375°F (190°C).
2. Core the apples and place them in a baking dish.
3. Sprinkle cinnamon evenly over the apples.
4. If using, fill the center of each apple with chopped nuts and drizzle with honey or agave nectar.
5. Bake for 20-25 minutes, or until the apples are tender.
6. Serve warm.

2. Greek Yogurt with Honey and Almonds

Ingredients:

- 1/2 cup low-fat Greek yogurt
- 1 tablespoon honey
- 1 tablespoon sliced almonds

Instructions:

1. Spoon the Greek yogurt into a bowl.
2. Drizzle honey over the yogurt.
3. Sprinkle sliced almonds on top.
4. Serve immediately.

3. Berry Parfait

Ingredients:

- 1/2 cup low-fat cottage cheese
- 1/4 cup fresh berries (such as strawberries, blueberries, or raspberries)
- 1 tablespoon chopped nuts (such as almonds or walnuts) (optional)
- 1 teaspoon honey or agave nectar (optional)

Instructions:

1. In a glass or bowl, layer the cottage cheese and fresh berries.
2. If using, sprinkle chopped nuts over the berries.

3. Drizzle with honey or agave nectar if desired.
4. Serve chilled.

4. Cocoa Banana Smoothie

Ingredients:

- 1 ripe banana
- 1 tablespoon unsweetened cocoa powder
- 1/2 cup low-fat milk or almond milk
- 1/4 teaspoon vanilla extract
- 1 teaspoon honey or agave nectar (optional)
- Ice cubes (optional)

Instructions:

1. Peel the banana and place it in a blender.
2. Add the cocoa powder, milk, vanilla extract, and honey or agave nectar if using.
3. If desired, add a few ice cubes to the blender for a colder smoothie.

4. Blend until smooth and creamy.
5. Pour into a glass and serve immediately.

5. Chia Seed Pudding with Berries

Ingredients:

- 2 tablespoons chia seeds
- 1/2 cup low-fat milk or almond milk
- 1/4 teaspoon vanilla extract
- 1 teaspoon honey or agave nectar (optional)
- 1/4 cup fresh berries (such as strawberries, blueberries, or raspberries)

Instructions:

1. In a bowl, mix together the chia seeds, milk, vanilla extract, and honey or agave nectar if using.
2. Cover and refrigerate for at least 2 hours, or overnight, until the pudding thickens.
3. Stir the pudding well before serving.

4. Serve topped with fresh berries.

6. Peanut Butter Banana Bites

Ingredients:

- 1 ripe banana, sliced
- 2 tablespoons natural peanut butter
- 1 tablespoon unsweetened shredded coconut (optional)
- 1 tablespoon chopped nuts (such as almonds or walnuts) (optional)

Instructions:

1. Spread peanut butter on each banana slice.
2. Sprinkle with shredded coconut and chopped nuts if desired.
3. Serve immediately.

7. Vanilla Yogurt with Sliced Peaches

Ingredients:

- 1/2 cup low-fat vanilla yogurt
- 1/2 fresh peach, sliced

- 1 tablespoon granola (optional)

Instructions:

1. Spoon the vanilla yogurt into a bowl.
2. Top with sliced peaches.
3. Sprinkle granola over the peaches if desired.
4. Serve chilled.

8. Cinnamon Baked Pears

Ingredients:

- 2 medium pears, halved and cored
- 1/2 teaspoon cinnamon
- 1 tablespoon chopped nuts (such as walnuts or almonds) (optional)
- 1 teaspoon honey or agave nectar (optional)

Instructions:

1. Preheat the oven to 375°F (190°C).
2. Place the pear halves in a baking dish, cut side up.

3. Sprinkle cinnamon evenly over the pears.
4. If using, fill the center of each pear half with chopped nuts and drizzle with honey or agave nectar.
5. Bake for 20-25 minutes, or until the pears are tender.
6. Serve warm.

9. Strawberry Frozen Yogurt Bark

Ingredients:

- 1 cup low-fat Greek yogurt
- 1/2 cup sliced strawberries
- 1 tablespoon honey or agave nectar (optional)
- 1 tablespoon unsweetened shredded coconut (optional)

Instructions:

1. Line a baking sheet with parchment paper.

2. Spread the Greek yogurt evenly onto the parchment paper, about 1/4 inch thick.

3. Sprinkle sliced strawberries over the yogurt.

4. Drizzle with honey or agave nectar if desired.

5. If using, sprinkle shredded coconut over the top.

6. Place the baking sheet in the freezer for at least 2 hours, or until the yogurt bark is firm.

7. Break the bark into pieces and serve immediately.

10. Chilled Chocolate Avocado Pudding

Ingredients:

- 1 ripe avocado
- 2 tablespoons unsweetened cocoa powder
- 2 tablespoons honey or agave nectar
- 1/4 cup low-fat milk or almond milk

- 1/2 teaspoon vanilla extract
- Pinch of salt

Instructions:

1. Scoop the avocado flesh into a blender or food processor.
2. Add the cocoa powder, honey or agave nectar, milk, vanilla extract, and salt.
3. Blend until smooth and creamy.
4. Refrigerate for at least 30 minutes before serving.
5. Serve chilled.

BEVERAGES RECIPES

1. Ginger Mint Tea

Ingredients:

- 1-inch piece of fresh ginger, peeled and sliced
- 2 cups water
- 1 tablespoon fresh mint leaves
- 1 teaspoon honey or agave nectar (optional)

- Lemon slice for garnish (optional)

Instructions:

1. Bring the water to a boil in a small pot.
2. Add the sliced ginger and reduce heat to a simmer.
3. Simmer for 10 minutes.
4. Add the fresh mint leaves and simmer for an additional 2 minutes.
5. Strain the tea into a cup.
6. Stir in honey or agave nectar if desired.
7. Garnish with a lemon slice if desired.
8. Serve warm.

2. Berry Smoothie

Ingredients:

- 1/2 cup low-fat Greek yogurt
- 1/2 cup unsweetened almond milk
- 1/2 cup fresh or frozen berries (such as strawberries, blueberries, or raspberries)

- 1 teaspoon honey or agave nectar (optional)
- Ice cubes (optional)

Instructions:

1. Combine the Greek yogurt, almond milk, berries, and honey or agave nectar (if using) in a blender.
2. Blend until smooth.
3. Add ice cubes if desired and blend again.
4. Pour into a glass and serve immediately.

3. Cucumber Mint Water

Ingredients:

- 1/2 cucumber, thinly sliced
- 1/4 cup fresh mint leaves
- 1 quart water
- Ice cubes

Instructions:

1. Place the cucumber slices and mint leaves in a pitcher.
2. Add the water and stir to combine.
3. Refrigerate for at least 1 hour to allow the flavors to infuse.
4. Serve chilled over ice cubes.

4. Vanilla Almond Milk Shake

Ingredients:

- 1 cup unsweetened almond milk
- 1/2 teaspoon vanilla extract
- 1 teaspoon honey or agave nectar (optional)
- 1/4 teaspoon ground cinnamon
- Ice cubes

Instructions:

1. Combine the almond milk, vanilla extract, honey or agave nectar (if using), and ground cinnamon in a blender.
2. Add ice cubes and blend until smooth.

3. Pour into a glass and serve immediately.

5. Lemon Ginger Water

Ingredients:

- 1 lemon, thinly sliced
- 1-inch piece of fresh ginger, peeled and thinly sliced
- 1 quart water
- Ice cubes

Instructions:

1. Place the lemon slices and ginger slices in a pitcher.
2. Add the water and stir to combine.
3. Refrigerate for at least 1 hour to allow the flavors to infuse.
4. Serve chilled over ice cubes.

HEALTHY AND APPETIZER RECIPES

1. Cucumber and Dill Yogurt Bites

Ingredients:

- 1 large cucumber, sliced into rounds
- 1/2 cup low-fat Greek yogurt
- 1 tablespoon fresh dill, finely chopped
- 1 teaspoon lemon juice
- Salt and pepper to taste

Instructions:

1. In a small bowl, mix the Greek yogurt, chopped dill, lemon juice, salt, and pepper.
2. Spoon a small amount of the yogurt mixture onto each cucumber slice.
3. Arrange the cucumber bites on a serving platter.
4. Serve chilled.

2. Caprese Skewers

Ingredients:

- 12 cherry tomatoes
- 12 small fresh mozzarella balls (bocconcini)
- 12 fresh basil leaves
- 1 tablespoon balsamic glaze (optional)

- Salt and pepper to taste

Instructions:

1. Thread one cherry tomato, one mozzarella ball, and one basil leaf onto each skewer.
2. Arrange the skewers on a serving platter.
3. Drizzle with balsamic glaze if desired.
4. Season with salt and pepper to taste.
5. Serve immediately.

3. Zucchini Roll-Ups with Hummus

Ingredients:

- 1 large zucchini, thinly sliced lengthwise
- 1/2 cup hummus (store-bought or homemade)
- 1/4 cup shredded carrots
- 1/4 cup chopped fresh parsley

Instructions:

1. Spread a thin layer of hummus over each zucchini slice.
2. Sprinkle shredded carrots and chopped parsley over the hummus.
3. Roll up the zucchini slices and secure with a toothpick.
4. Arrange the roll-ups on a serving platter.
5. Serve immediately.

4. Avocado Deviled Eggs

Ingredients:

- 4 hard-boiled eggs, peeled and halved
- 1 ripe avocado
- 1 teaspoon lemon juice
- Salt and pepper to taste
- Paprika for garnish (optional)

Instructions:

1. Remove the yolks from the hard-boiled eggs and place them in a bowl.

2. Add the avocado and lemon juice to the bowl.
3. Mash the yolks and avocado together until smooth.
4. Season with salt and pepper to taste.
5. Spoon the avocado mixture into the egg white halves.
6. Garnish with paprika if desired.
7. Serve immediately.

5. Baked Zucchini Chips

Ingredients:

- 1 large zucchini, thinly sliced into rounds
- 1 tablespoon olive oil
- 1/2 teaspoon garlic powder
- 1/2 teaspoon paprika
- Salt and pepper to taste

Instructions:

1. Preheat the oven to 375°F (190°C) and line a baking sheet with parchment paper.

2. In a bowl, toss the zucchini slices with olive oil, garlic powder, paprika, salt, and pepper.
3. Arrange the zucchini slices in a single layer on the prepared baking sheet.
4. Bake for 20-25 minutes, or until the zucchini chips are crispy and golden brown.
5. Allow to cool slightly before serving.

30DAY MEAL PLAN

Day 1

Breakfast:

- Smooth Banana Oatmeal
  - Ingredients: 1/2 cup oats, 1 cup low-fat milk or almond milk, 1/2 ripe banana (mashed), 1 tsp cinnamon
  - Instructions: Cook oats with milk, stir in mashed banana and cinnamon.

Lunch:

- Chicken and Rice Soup
  - Ingredients: 1/2 cup cooked chicken breast (shredded), 1/2 cup cooked white rice, 1 cup low-sodium chicken broth, 1/4 cup diced carrots, 1/4 cup diced celery
  - Instructions: Combine all ingredients in a pot and heat until vegetables are tender.

Snack:

- Greek Yogurt with Honey
  - Ingredients: 1/2 cup low-fat Greek yogurt, 1 tsp honey

Dinner:

- Baked Salmon with Mashed Sweet Potatoes
  - Ingredients: 1 salmon fillet, 1 cup mashed sweet potatoes, 1 tsp olive oil, salt and pepper to taste

o Instructions: Bake salmon at 375°F for 15-20 minutes. Serve with mashed sweet potatoes.

Day 2

Breakfast:

- Scrambled Eggs with Spinach
    - o Ingredients: 2 eggs, 1/2 cup fresh spinach, 1 tsp olive oil
    - o Instructions: Scramble eggs with spinach and olive oil.

Lunch:

- Turkey and Cheese Roll-Ups
    - o Ingredients: 2 slices low-sodium deli turkey, 2 slices low-fat cheese, 1/4 cup baby spinach
    - o Instructions: Roll up turkey and cheese with spinach inside.

Snack:

- Cottage Cheese with Pineapple

- o Ingredients: 1/2 cup low-fat cottage cheese, 1/4 cup diced pineapple

Dinner:

- Baked Chicken with Steamed Zucchini
  - o Ingredients: 1 chicken breast, 1 cup steamed zucchini, 1 tsp olive oil, salt and pepper to taste
  - o Instructions: Bake chicken at 375°F for 25-30 minutes. Serve with steamed zucchini.

Day 3

Breakfast:

- Vanilla Almond Milk Shake
  - o Ingredients: 1 cup unsweetened almond milk, 1/2 tsp vanilla extract, 1 tsp honey, ice cubes
  - o Instructions: Blend all ingredients until smooth.

Lunch:

- Tuna Salad Lettuce Wraps
  - Ingredients: 1 can (5 oz) tuna, 1 tbsp low-fat mayonnaise, 1 tsp Dijon mustard, 1/4 cup diced celery, 4 large lettuce leaves
  - Instructions: Mix tuna, mayonnaise, mustard, and celery. Spoon onto lettuce leaves and wrap.

Snack:

- Sliced Apples with Almond Butter
  - Ingredients: 1 small apple (sliced), 1 tbsp almond butter

Dinner:

- Shrimp and Rice Bowl
  - Ingredients: 1 cup cooked white rice, 1/2 pound shrimp (peeled and deveined), 1 tbsp olive oil, 1/2 cup diced zucchini, 1 tbsp low-sodium soy sauce, 1 tbsp lemon juice

- Instructions: Cook shrimp and
    zucchini in olive oil, add soy
    sauce and lemon juice, serve
    over rice.

Day 4

Breakfast:

- Berry Parfait
  - Ingredients: 1/2 cup low-fat
    Greek yogurt, 1/4 cup fresh
    berries, 1 tbsp chopped nuts
  - Instructions: Layer yogurt,
    berries, and nuts in a bowl.

Lunch:

- Mild Fish Curry
  - Ingredients: 1 white fish fillet
    (cut into chunks), 1 tbsp olive
    oil, 1/2 small onion (chopped), 1
    clove garlic (minced), 1/2 cup
    low-sodium chicken broth, 1/2
    cup light coconut milk, 1 tsp

turmeric, 1/2 tsp cumin, salt and pepper to taste
  - Instructions: Cook onion and garlic in olive oil, add spices, broth, and coconut milk. Add fish and simmer until cooked.

Snack:

- Cucumber Mint Water
  - Ingredients: 1/2 cucumber (sliced), 1/4 cup fresh mint leaves, 1 quart water
  - Instructions: Combine all ingredients in a pitcher and refrigerate.

Dinner:

- Turkey Meatballs with Mashed Potatoes
  - Ingredients: 1/2 pound ground turkey, 1/4 cup breadcrumbs, 1 egg, 1/4 cup grated Parmesan, 2 medium potatoes (peeled and diced), 1/4 cup low-fat milk

- ○ Instructions: Mix turkey, breadcrumbs, egg, and Parmesan, form into meatballs, bake at 375°F for 20-25 minutes. Boil and mash potatoes with milk.

Day 5

Breakfast:

- Peanut Butter Banana Smoothie
  - ○ Ingredients: 1 ripe banana, 1 tbsp peanut butter, 1 cup low-fat milk, ice cubes
  - ○ Instructions: Blend all ingredients until smooth.

Lunch:

- Avocado and Egg Salad
  - ○ Ingredients: 1 ripe avocado, 2 hard-boiled eggs, 1 tsp lemon juice, salt and pepper to taste

  - Instructions: Mash avocado and mix with chopped hard-boiled eggs and lemon juice.

Snack:

- Cottage Cheese with Sliced Peaches
  - Ingredients: 1/2 cup low-fat cottage cheese, 1/2 fresh peach (sliced)

Dinner:

- Baked Cod with Steamed Carrots
  - Ingredients: 1 cod fillet, 1 cup steamed carrots, 1 tsp olive oil, salt and pepper to taste
  - Instructions: Bake cod at 375°F for 15-20 minutes. Serve with steamed carrots.

Day 6

Breakfast:

- Berry Smoothie

- Ingredients: 1/2 cup low-fat Greek yogurt, 1/2 cup unsweetened almond milk, 1/2 cup fresh or frozen berries, 1 tsp honey
  - Instructions: Blend all ingredients until smooth.

Lunch:

- Chicken and Butternut Squash Puree
  - Ingredients: 1 boneless chicken breast, 1 cup butternut squash (cubed), 1 tbsp olive oil, 1/4 cup low-sodium chicken broth
  - Instructions: Bake chicken at 375°F for 25-30 minutes. Steam squash and blend with broth until smooth.

Snack:

- Greek Yogurt with Berries
  - Ingredients: 1/2 cup low-fat Greek yogurt, 1/4 cup fresh berries

Dinner:

- Tofu and Carrot Ginger Soup
    - Ingredients: 1/2 block firm tofu (cubed), 2 large carrots (diced), 1 small onion (chopped), 1 clove garlic (minced), 1 tsp grated ginger, 3 cups low-sodium vegetable broth
    - Instructions: Cook onion, garlic, and ginger in olive oil, add carrots and broth, simmer until carrots are tender, add tofu and heat through.

Day 7

Breakfast:

- Chia Seed Pudding
    - Ingredients: 2 tbsp chia seeds, 1/2 cup low-fat milk, 1/4 tsp vanilla extract, 1 tsp honey, 1/4 cup fresh berries

- Instructions: Mix chia seeds, milk, vanilla, and honey, refrigerate until thickened. Top with berries before serving.

Lunch:

- Mild Fish Curry
  - Ingredients: 1 white fish fillet (cut into chunks), 1 tbsp olive oil, 1/2 small onion (chopped), 1 clove garlic (minced), 1/2 cup low-sodium chicken broth, 1/2 cup light coconut milk, 1 tsp turmeric, 1/2 tsp cumin, salt and pepper to taste
  - Instructions: Cook onion and garlic in olive oil, add spices, broth, and coconut milk. Add fish and simmer until cooked.

Snack:

- Vanilla Yogurt with Sliced Peaches

- ○ Ingredients: 1/2 cup low-fat vanilla yogurt, 1/2 fresh peach (sliced)

Dinner:

- Baked Turkey Meatballs with Mashed Potatoes
  - ○ Ingredients: 1/2 pound ground turkey, 1/4 cup breadcrumbs, 1 egg, 1/4 cup grated Parmesan, 2 medium potatoes (peeled and diced), 1/4 cup low-fat milk
  - ○ Instructions: Mix turkey, breadcrumbs, egg, and Parmesan, form into meatballs, bake at 375°F for 20-25 minutes. Boil and mash potatoes with milk.

Day 8

Breakfast:

- Smooth Banana Oatmeal

- Ingredients: 1/2 cup oats, 1 cup low-fat milk or almond milk, 1/2 ripe banana (mashed), 1 tsp cinnamon
  - Instructions: Cook oats with milk, stir in mashed banana and cinnamon.

Lunch:

- Chicken and Rice Soup
  - Ingredients: 1/2 cup cooked chicken breast (shredded), 1/2 cup cooked white rice, 1 cup low-sodium chicken broth, 1/4 cup diced carrots, 1/4 cup diced celery
  - Instructions: Combine all ingredients in a pot and heat until vegetables are tender.

Snack:

- Greek Yogurt with Honey
  - Ingredients: 1/2 cup low-fat Greek yogurt, 1 tsp honey

Dinner:

- Baked Salmon with Mashed Sweet Potatoes
    - Ingredients: 1 salmon fillet, 1 cup mashed sweet potatoes, 1 tsp olive oil, salt and pepper to taste
    - Instructions: Bake salmon at 375°F for 15-20 minutes. Serve with mashed sweet potatoes.

Day 9

Breakfast:

- Scrambled Eggs with Spinach
    - Ingredients: 2 eggs, 1/2 cup fresh spinach, 1 tsp olive oil
    - Instructions: Scramble eggs with spinach and olive oil.

Lunch:

- Turkey and Cheese Roll-Ups

- Ingredients: 2 slices low-sodium deli turkey, 2 slices low-fat cheese, 1/4 cup baby spinach
  - Instructions: Roll up turkey and cheese with spinach inside.

Snack:

- Cottage Cheese with Pineapple
  - Ingredients: 1/2 cup low-fat cottage cheese, 1/4 cup diced pineapple

Dinner:

- Baked Chicken with Steamed Zucchini
  - Ingredients: 1 chicken breast, 1 cup steamed zucchini, 1 tsp olive oil, salt and pepper to taste
  - Instructions: Bake chicken at 375°F for 25-30 minutes. Serve with steamed zucchini.

Day 10

Breakfast:

- Vanilla Almond Milk Shake
    - Ingredients: 1 cup unsweetened almond milk, 1/2 tsp vanilla extract, 1 tsp honey, ice cubes
    - Instructions: Blend all ingredients until smooth.

Lunch:

- Tuna Salad Lettuce Wraps
    - Ingredients: 1 can (5 oz) tuna, 1 tbsp low-fat mayonnaise, 1 tsp Dijon mustard, 1/4 cup diced celery, 4 large lettuce leaves
    - Instructions: Mix tuna, mayonnaise, mustard, and celery. Spoon onto lettuce leaves and wrap.

Snack:

- Sliced Apples with Almond Butter
    - Ingredients: 1 small apple (sliced), 1 tbsp almond butter

Dinner:

- Shrimp and Rice Bowl
    - Ingredients: 1 cup cooked white rice, 1/2 pound shrimp (peeled and deveined), 1 tbsp olive oil, 1/2 cup diced zucchini, 1 tbsp low-sodium soy sauce, 1 tbsp lemon juice
    - Instructions: Cook shrimp and zucchini in olive oil, add soy sauce and lemon juice, serve over rice.

Day 11

Breakfast:

- Berry Parfait
    - Ingredients: 1/2 cup low-fat Greek yogurt, 1/4 cup fresh berries, 1 tbsp chopped nuts
    - Instructions: Layer yogurt, berries, and nuts in a bowl.

Lunch:

- Mild Fish Curry

o Ingredients: 1 white fish fillet (cut into chunks), 1 tbsp olive oil, 1/2 small onion (chopped), 1 clove garlic (minced), 1/2 cup low-sodium chicken broth, 1/2 cup light coconut milk, 1 tsp turmeric, 1/2 tsp cumin, salt and pepper to taste
o Instructions: Cook onion and garlic in olive oil, add spices, broth, and coconut milk. Add fish and simmer until cooked.

Snack:

- Cucumber Mint Water
  - o Ingredients: 1/2 cucumber (sliced), 1/4 cup fresh mint leaves, 1 quart water
  - o Instructions: Combine all ingredients in a pitcher and refrigerate.

Dinner:

- Turkey Meatballs with Mashed Potatoes
    - Ingredients: 1/2 pound ground turkey, 1/4 cup breadcrumbs, 1 egg, 1/4 cup grated Parmesan, 2 medium potatoes (peeled and diced), 1/4 cup low-fat milk
    - Instructions: Mix turkey, breadcrumbs, egg, and Parmesan, form into meatballs, bake at 375°F for 20-25 minutes. Boil and mash potatoes with milk.

Day 12

Breakfast:

- Peanut Butter Banana Smoothie
    - Ingredients: 1 ripe banana, 1 tbsp peanut butter, 1 cup low-fat milk, ice cubes
    - Instructions: Blend all ingredients until smooth.

Lunch:

- Avocado and Egg Salad
  - Ingredients: 1 ripe avocado, 2 hard-boiled eggs, 1 tsp lemon juice, salt and pepper to taste
  - Instructions: Mash avocado and mix with chopped hard-boiled eggs and lemon juice.

Snack:

- Cottage Cheese with Sliced Peaches
  - Ingredients: 1/2 cup low-fat cottage cheese, 1/2 fresh peach (sliced)

Dinner:

- Baked Cod with Steamed Carrots
  - Ingredients: 1 cod fillet, 1 cup steamed carrots, 1 tsp olive oil, salt and pepper to taste
  - Instructions: Bake cod at 375°F for 15-20 minutes. Serve with steamed carrots.

Day 13

Breakfast:

- Berry Smoothie
  - Ingredients: 1/2 cup low-fat Greek yogurt, 1/2 cup unsweetened almond milk, 1/2 cup fresh or frozen berries, 1 tsp honey
  - Instructions: Blend all ingredients until smooth.

Lunch:

- Chicken and Butternut Squash Puree
  - Ingredients: 1 boneless chicken breast, 1 cup butternut squash (cubed), 1 tbsp olive oil, 1/4 cup low-sodium chicken broth
  - Instructions: Bake chicken at 375°F for 25-30 minutes. Steam squash and blend with broth until smooth.

Snack:

- Greek Yogurt with Berries
  - Ingredients: 1/2 cup low-fat Greek yogurt, 1/4 cup fresh berries

Dinner:

- Tofu and Carrot Ginger Soup
  - Ingredients: 1/2 block firm tofu (cubed), 2 large carrots (diced), 1 small onion (chopped), 1 clove garlic (minced), 1 tsp grated ginger, 3 cups low-sodium vegetable broth
  - Instructions: Cook onion, garlic, and ginger in olive oil, add carrots and broth, simmer until carrots are tender, add tofu and heat through.

Day 14

Breakfast:

- Chia Seed Pudding

- Ingredients: 2 tbsp chia seeds, 1/2 cup low-fat milk, 1/4 tsp vanilla extract, 1 tsp honey, 1/4 cup fresh berries
  - Instructions: Mix chia seeds, milk, vanilla, and honey, refrigerate until thickened. Top with berries before serving.

Lunch:

- Mild Fish Curry
  - Ingredients: 1 white fish fillet (cut into chunks), 1 tbsp olive oil, 1/2 small onion (chopped), 1 clove garlic (minced), 1/2 cup low-sodium chicken broth, 1/2 cup light coconut milk, 1 tsp turmeric, 1/2 tsp cumin, salt and pepper to taste
  - Instructions: Cook onion and garlic in olive oil, add spices, broth, and coconut milk. Add fish and simmer until cooked.

Snack:

- Vanilla Yogurt with Sliced Peaches
    - Ingredients: 1/2 cup low-fat vanilla yogurt, 1/2 fresh peach (sliced)

Dinner:

- Baked Turkey Meatballs with Mashed Potatoes
    - Ingredients: 1/2 pound ground turkey, 1/4 cup breadcrumbs, 1 egg, 1/4 cup grated Parmesan, 2 medium potatoes (peeled and diced), 1/4 cup low-fat milk
    - Instructions: Mix turkey, breadcrumbs, egg, and Parmesan, form into meatballs, bake at 375°F for 20-25 minutes. Boil and mash potatoes with milk.

Day 15

Breakfast:

- Apple Cinnamon Oatmeal
    - Ingredients: 1/2 cup oats, 1 cup low-fat milk or almond milk, 1/2 apple (peeled and finely diced), 1 tsp cinnamon
    - Instructions: Cook oats with milk, stir in diced apple and cinnamon, cook until apple is tender.

Lunch:

- Grilled Chicken and Quinoa Salad
    - Ingredients: 1/2 cup cooked quinoa, 1 grilled chicken breast (sliced), 1/2 cup diced cucumber, 1/4 cup diced red bell pepper, 1 tbsp olive oil, 1 tbsp lemon juice, salt and pepper to taste
    - Instructions: Mix quinoa, chicken, cucumber, and bell pepper. Dress with olive oil and lemon juice, season with salt and pepper.

Snack:

- Smooth Peanut Butter Banana
  - Ingredients: 1 small banana, 1 tbsp smooth peanut butter

Dinner:

- Baked Tilapia with Steamed Broccoli
  - Ingredients: 1 tilapia fillet, 1 cup steamed broccoli, 1 tsp olive oil, salt and pepper to taste
  - Instructions: Bake tilapia at 375°F for 15-20 minutes. Serve with steamed broccoli.

Day 16

Breakfast:

- Greek Yogurt with Berries and Honey
  - Ingredients: 1/2 cup low-fat Greek yogurt, 1/4 cup fresh berries, 1 tsp honey
  - Instructions: Top yogurt with berries and honey.

Lunch:

- Turkey and Avocado Wrap
  - Ingredients: 1 whole wheat tortilla, 2 slices low-sodium deli turkey, 1/2 avocado (sliced), 1/4 cup shredded lettuce
  - Instructions: Layer turkey, avocado, and lettuce on tortilla, roll up.

Snack:

- Cottage Cheese with Melon
  - Ingredients: 1/2 cup low-fat cottage cheese, 1/4 cup diced melon (such as cantaloupe or honeydew)

Dinner:

- Beef and Vegetable Stir-Fry
  - Ingredients: 1/2 cup lean beef strips, 1/2 cup broccoli florets, 1/2 cup sliced carrots, 1 tbsp

low-sodium soy sauce, 1 tbsp olive oil
- Instructions: Stir-fry beef and vegetables in olive oil, add soy sauce.

Day 17

Breakfast:

- Smoothie with Spinach and Berries
    - Ingredients: 1/2 cup low-fat Greek yogurt, 1/2 cup unsweetened almond milk, 1/2 cup fresh or frozen berries, 1/2 cup fresh spinach, 1 tsp honey
    - Instructions: Blend all ingredients until smooth.

Lunch:

- Chicken and Avocado Salad
    - Ingredients: 1/2 cup cooked chicken breast (diced), 1/2 avocado (diced), 1/4 cup cherry tomatoes (halved), 1 tbsp olive

oil, 1 tbsp lemon juice, salt and pepper to taste
- ○ Instructions: Mix chicken, avocado, and tomatoes. Dress with olive oil and lemon juice, season with salt and pepper.

Snack:

- Sliced Cucumbers with Hummus
  - ○ Ingredients: 1/2 cucumber (sliced), 1/4 cup hummus

Dinner:

- Baked Pork Chops with Sweet Potato Mash
  - ○ Ingredients: 1 pork chop, 1 cup mashed sweet potatoes, 1 tsp olive oil, salt and pepper to taste
  - ○ Instructions: Bake pork chop at 375°F for 25-30 minutes. Serve with mashed sweet potatoes.

Day 18

Breakfast:

- Vanilla Chia Seed Pudding
  - Ingredients: 2 tbsp chia seeds, 1/2 cup low-fat milk, 1/4 tsp vanilla extract, 1 tsp honey, 1/4 cup fresh berries
  - Instructions: Mix chia seeds, milk, vanilla, and honey, refrigerate until thickened. Top with berries before serving.

Lunch:

- Shrimp and Avocado Salad
  - Ingredients: 1/2 cup cooked shrimp, 1/2 avocado (diced), 1/4 cup cherry tomatoes (halved), 1 tbsp olive oil, 1 tbsp lime juice, salt and pepper to taste
  - Instructions: Mix shrimp, avocado, and tomatoes. Dress with olive oil and lime juice, season with salt and pepper.

Snack:

- Greek Yogurt with Sliced Strawberries
  - Ingredients: 1/2 cup low-fat Greek yogurt, 1/4 cup sliced strawberries

Dinner:

- Lemon Herb Chicken with Steamed Green Beans
  - Ingredients: 1 chicken breast, 1 tbsp lemon juice, 1 tsp olive oil, 1 tsp dried herbs (such as thyme or rosemary), 1 cup steamed green beans
  - Instructions: Marinate chicken in lemon juice, olive oil, and herbs, bake at 375°F for 25-30 minutes. Serve with steamed green beans.

Day 19

Breakfast:

- Smoothie with Mango and Pineapple

- Ingredients: 1/2 cup low-fat Greek yogurt, 1/2 cup unsweetened almond milk, 1/2 cup fresh or frozen mango, 1/2 cup fresh or frozen pineapple
  - Instructions: Blend all ingredients until smooth.

Lunch:

- Grilled Turkey and Vegetable Skewers
  - Ingredients: 1/2 cup turkey breast (cubed), 1/2 cup diced bell peppers, 1/2 cup diced zucchini, 1 tbsp olive oil, salt and pepper to taste
  - Instructions: Thread turkey and vegetables onto skewers, brush with olive oil, season with salt and pepper, grill until cooked.

Snack:

- Cottage Cheese with Berries

     ○ Ingredients: 1/2 cup low-fat cottage cheese, 1/4 cup fresh berries

Dinner:

- Baked Salmon with Asparagus
  - ○ Ingredients: 1 salmon fillet, 1 cup asparagus spears, 1 tsp olive oil, salt and pepper to taste
  - ○ Instructions: Bake salmon at 375°F for 15-20 minutes. Serve with steamed asparagus.

Day 20

Breakfast:

- Peach Smoothie
  - ○ Ingredients: 1/2 cup low-fat Greek yogurt, 1/2 cup unsweetened almond milk, 1/2 cup fresh or frozen peach slices, 1 tsp honey
  - ○ Instructions: Blend all ingredients until smooth.

Lunch:

- Chicken and Quinoa Bowl
  - Ingredients: 1/2 cup cooked quinoa, 1/2 cup cooked chicken breast (diced), 1/4 cup diced cucumber, 1/4 cup diced tomatoes, 1 tbsp olive oil, 1 tbsp lemon juice, salt and pepper to taste
  - Instructions: Mix quinoa, chicken, cucumber, and tomatoes. Dress with olive oil and lemon juice, season with salt and pepper.

Snack:

- Sliced Apples with Almond Butter
  - Ingredients: 1 small apple (sliced), 1 tbsp almond butter

Dinner:

- Baked Cod with Steamed Broccoli

- o Ingredients: 1 cod fillet, 1 cup steamed broccoli, 1 tsp olive oil, salt and pepper to taste
  - o Instructions: Bake cod at 375°F for 15-20 minutes. Serve with steamed broccoli.

Day 21

Breakfast:

- Banana Oatmeal Smoothie
  - o Ingredients: 1 ripe banana, 1/2 cup cooked oats, 1 cup low-fat milk or almond milk, 1 tsp cinnamon
  - o Instructions: Blend all ingredients until smooth.

Lunch:

- Tuna and Avocado Salad
  - o Ingredients: 1 can (5 oz) tuna, 1/2 avocado (diced), 1/4 cup cherry tomatoes (halved), 1 tbsp

olive oil, 1 tbsp lemon juice, salt and pepper to taste
  - Instructions: Mix tuna, avocado, and tomatoes. Dress with olive oil and lemon juice, season with salt and pepper.

Snack:

- Greek Yogurt with Honey and Nuts
  - Ingredients: 1/2 cup low-fat Greek yogurt, 1 tsp honey, 1 tbsp chopped nuts

Dinner:

- Chicken Stir-Fry with Rice
  - Ingredients: 1 chicken breast (sliced), 1/2 cup sliced carrots, 1/2 cup broccoli florets, 1 tbsp low-sodium soy sauce, 1 tbsp olive oil, 1/2 cup cooked white rice
  - Instructions: Stir-fry chicken and vegetables in olive oil, add soy sauce, serve over rice.

Day 22

Breakfast:

- Blueberry Almond Smoothie
    - Ingredients: 1/2 cup low-fat Greek yogurt, 1/2 cup unsweetened almond milk, 1/2 cup fresh or frozen blueberries, 1 tbsp almond butter
    - Instructions: Blend all ingredients until smooth.

Lunch:

- Chicken and Spinach Salad
    - Ingredients: 1/2 cup cooked chicken breast (diced), 1 cup fresh spinach, 1/4 cup cherry tomatoes (halved), 1 tbsp olive oil, 1 tbsp balsamic vinegar, salt and pepper to taste
    - Instructions: Mix spinach, chicken, and tomatoes. Dress with olive oil and balsamic

vinegar, season with salt and pepper.

Snack:

- Greek Yogurt with Honey and Cinnamon
  - Ingredients: 1/2 cup low-fat Greek yogurt, 1 tsp honey, 1/2 tsp cinnamon

Dinner:

- Baked Haddock with Steamed Carrots
  - Ingredients: 1 haddock fillet, 1 cup steamed carrots, 1 tsp olive oil, salt and pepper to taste
  - Instructions: Bake haddock at 375°F for 15-20 minutes. Serve with steamed carrots.

Day 23

Breakfast:

- Strawberry Banana Smoothie

- ○ Ingredients: 1/2 cup low-fat Greek yogurt, 1/2 cup unsweetened almond milk, 1/2 cup fresh or frozen strawberries, 1/2 ripe banana
  - ○ Instructions: Blend all ingredients until smooth.

Lunch:

- Turkey and Cucumber Wrap
  - ○ Ingredients: 1 whole wheat tortilla, 2 slices low-sodium deli turkey, 1/2 cucumber (sliced), 1 tbsp hummus
  - ○ Instructions: Spread hummus on tortilla, layer turkey and cucumber, roll up.

Snack:

- Cottage Cheese with Pineapple
  - ○ Ingredients: 1/2 cup low-fat cottage cheese, 1/4 cup diced pineapple

Dinner:

- Grilled Chicken with Steamed Green Beans
    - Ingredients: 1 chicken breast, 1 cup steamed green beans, 1 tsp olive oil, salt and pepper to taste
    - Instructions: Grill chicken breast. Serve with steamed green beans.

Day 24

Breakfast:

- Mango Coconut Smoothie
    - Ingredients: 1/2 cup low-fat Greek yogurt, 1/2 cup unsweetened coconut milk, 1/2 cup fresh or frozen mango, 1 tbsp shredded coconut
    - Instructions: Blend all ingredients until smooth.

Lunch:

- Quinoa and Vegetable Bowl
  - Ingredients: 1/2 cup cooked quinoa, 1/4 cup diced cucumber, 1/4 cup diced bell pepper, 1/4 cup cherry tomatoes, 1 tbsp olive oil, 1 tbsp lemon juice, salt and pepper to taste
  - Instructions: Mix quinoa and vegetables. Dress with olive oil and lemon juice, season with salt and pepper.

Snack:

- Greek Yogurt with Blueberries
  - Ingredients: 1/2 cup low-fat Greek yogurt, 1/4 cup fresh blueberries

Dinner:

- Baked Cod with Mashed Sweet Potatoes
  - Ingredients: 1 cod fillet, 1 cup mashed sweet potatoes, 1 tsp olive oil, salt and pepper to taste

o Instructions: Bake cod at 375°F for 15-20 minutes. Serve with mashed sweet potatoes.

Day 25

Breakfast:

- Apple Cinnamon Smoothie
  - Ingredients: 1/2 cup low-fat Greek yogurt, 1/2 cup unsweetened almond milk, 1/2 apple (peeled and chopped), 1 tsp cinnamon
  - Instructions: Blend all ingredients until smooth.

Lunch:

- Chicken Avocado Wrap
  - Ingredients: 1 whole wheat tortilla, 1/2 cup cooked chicken breast (diced), 1/2 avocado (sliced), 1/4 cup shredded lettuce

- o Instructions: Layer chicken, avocado, and lettuce on tortilla, roll up.

Snack:

- Cottage Cheese with Melon
    - o Ingredients: 1/2 cup low-fat cottage cheese, 1/4 cup diced melon (such as cantaloupe or honeydew)

Dinner:

- Baked Salmon with Steamed Broccoli
    - o Ingredients: 1 salmon fillet, 1 cup steamed broccoli, 1 tsp olive oil, salt and pepper to taste
    - o Instructions: Bake salmon at 375°F for 15-20 minutes. Serve with steamed broccoli.

Day 26

Breakfast:

- Peach Smoothie
  - Ingredients: 1/2 cup low-fat Greek yogurt, 1/2 cup unsweetened almond milk, 1/2 cup fresh or frozen peach slices, 1 tsp honey
  - Instructions: Blend all ingredients until smooth.

Lunch:

- Shrimp and Avocado Salad
  - Ingredients: 1/2 cup cooked shrimp, 1/2 avocado (diced), 1/4 cup cherry tomatoes (halved), 1 tbsp olive oil, 1 tbsp lime juice, salt and pepper to taste
  - Instructions: Mix shrimp, avocado, and tomatoes. Dress with olive oil and lime juice, season with salt and pepper.

Snack:

- Greek Yogurt with Sliced Peaches

- Ingredients: 1/2 cup low-fat Greek yogurt, 1/2 fresh peach (sliced)

Dinner:

- Baked Chicken with Steamed Carrots
  - Ingredients: 1 chicken breast, 1 cup steamed carrots, 1 tsp olive oil, salt and pepper to taste
  - Instructions: Bake chicken at 375°F for 25-30 minutes. Serve with steamed carrots.

Day 27

Breakfast:

- Spinach Banana Smoothie
  - Ingredients: 1/2 cup low-fat Greek yogurt, 1/2 cup unsweetened almond milk, 1/2 ripe banana, 1/2 cup fresh spinach
  - Instructions: Blend all ingredients until smooth.

Lunch:

- Tuna and Avocado Salad
    - Ingredients: 1 can (5 oz) tuna, 1/2 avocado (diced), 1/4 cup cherry tomatoes (halved), 1 tbsp olive oil, 1 tbsp lemon juice, salt and pepper to taste
    - Instructions: Mix tuna, avocado, and tomatoes. Dress with olive oil and lemon juice, season with salt and pepper.

Snack:

- Cottage Cheese with Sliced Strawberries
    - Ingredients: 1/2 cup low-fat cottage cheese, 1/4 cup sliced strawberries

Dinner:

- Grilled Turkey Burgers with Steamed Zucchini

- o Ingredients: 1 turkey burger patty, 1 whole wheat bun, 1 cup steamed zucchini, 1 tsp olive oil, salt and pepper to taste
  - o Instructions: Grill turkey burger, serve on whole wheat bun with steamed zucchini.

Day 28

Breakfast:

- Vanilla Almond Smoothie
  - o Ingredients: 1/2 cup low-fat Greek yogurt, 1/2 cup unsweetened almond milk, 1/2 tsp vanilla extract, 1 tbsp almond butter
  - o Instructions: Blend all ingredients until smooth.

Lunch:

- Chicken and Quinoa Salad
  - o Ingredients: 1/2 cup cooked quinoa, 1/2 cup cooked chicken

breast (diced), 1/4 cup diced cucumber, 1/4 cup diced bell pepper, 1 tbsp olive oil, 1 tbsp lemon juice, salt and pepper to taste
  - Instructions: Mix quinoa, chicken, and vegetables. Dress with olive oil and lemon juice, season with salt and pepper.

Snack:

- Greek Yogurt with Honey and Almonds
  - Ingredients: 1/2 cup low-fat Greek yogurt, 1 tsp honey, 1 tbsp chopped almonds

Dinner:

- Baked Tilapia with Mashed Potatoes
  - Ingredients: 1 tilapia fillet, 1 cup mashed potatoes, 1 tsp olive oil, salt and pepper to taste

o Instructions: Bake tilapia at 375°F for 15-20 minutes. Serve with mashed potatoes.

Day 29

Breakfast:

- Berry Smoothie
    - Ingredients: 1/2 cup low-fat Greek yogurt, 1/2 cup unsweetened almond milk, 1/2 cup fresh or frozen berries, 1 tsp honey
    - Instructions: Blend all ingredients until smooth.

Lunch:

- Turkey and Cheese Roll-Ups
    - Ingredients: 2 slices low-sodium deli turkey, 2 slices low-fat cheese, 1/4 cup baby spinach
    - Instructions: Roll up turkey and cheese with spinach inside.

Snack:

- Cottage Cheese with Pineapple
    - Ingredients: 1/2 cup low-fat cottage cheese, 1/4 cup diced pineapple

Dinner:

- Grilled Chicken with Steamed Green Beans
    - Ingredients: 1 chicken breast, 1 cup steamed green beans, 1 tsp olive oil, salt and pepper to taste
    - Instructions: Grill chicken breast. Serve with steamed green beans.

Day 30

Breakfast:

- Pineapple Coconut Smoothie
    - Ingredients: 1/2 cup low-fat Greek yogurt, 1/2 cup unsweetened coconut milk, 1/2

cup fresh or frozen pineapple, 1 tbsp shredded coconut

- ○ Instructions: Blend all ingredients until smooth.

Lunch:

- Shrimp and Avocado Salad
  - ○ Ingredients: 1/2 cup cooked shrimp, 1/2 avocado (diced), 1/4 cup cherry tomatoes (halved), 1 tbsp olive oil, 1 tbsp lime juice, salt and pepper to taste
  - ○ Instructions: Mix shrimp, avocado, and tomatoes. Dress with olive oil and lime juice, season with salt and pepper.

Snack:

- Greek Yogurt with Sliced Peaches
  - ○ Ingredients: 1/2 cup low-fat Greek yogurt, 1/2 fresh peach (sliced)

Dinner:

- Baked Cod with Steamed Broccoli
  - Ingredients: 1 cod fillet, 1 cup steamed broccoli, 1 tsp olive oil, salt and pepper to taste
  - Instructions: Bake cod at 375°F for 15-20 minutes. Serve with steamed broccoli.

CONCLUSION

Discover the essential guide to managing diabetic gastroparesis with our comprehensive diet cookbook for beginners. Packed with easy-to-follow recipes, this cookbook offers a variety of delicious and nutritious meals tailored to support digestive health and regulate blood sugar levels. Whether you're newly diagnosed or seeking fresh ideas for managing your condition, this cookbook provides the tools and inspiration you need to embrace a healthy lifestyle. Say goodbye to uncertainty and hello to flavorful meals designed to nourish and satisfy. Order your copy today and take the first step towards a happier, healthier you!"

THE END

www.ingramcontent.com/pod-product-compliance
Lightning Source LLC
Chambersburg PA
CBHW071016250726
48653CB00005B/1629